Healthy Body, Healthy Mind,
Healthy Life

Part I

Nutrition

JOE BOONE

CSCS, CISSN

COPYRIGHT & DISCLAIMER

TABLE OF CONTENTS

INTRODUCTION

In *Healthy Body, Healthy Mind, Healthy Life Part I: Nutrition* we look at the many aspects of the diet including macronutrients, micronutrients, water, alcohol, metabolism, and even the cheat day. All of these topics are important for establishing that foundation of knowledge which is needed when it comes to understanding what you are putting into your body.

Too often people sensationalize ideas around nutrition and the big picture loses its value. Usually you see this as a diet or supplement that people are claiming is the best. The problem is that most people don't understand the basics and the ideas that are thrown around on social media become the focus rather than the solid science that backs nutrition. Yes, there will always be manipulations of dietary styles to provide some novel attempt at enhancing goals like fat loss, mass gain, performance, etc. but these attempts are all centered out of the big picture of nutrition.

Understanding the foundational information can aid you in attaining whatever your goal is without being sucked into the pseudo-science and people's belief systems that surround how they eat. What you eat and how you do it should be based on the evidence, your goals, what you like, and even trial and error.

I hope that what I have given you in the following text allows you to see nutrition in a clearer scope. I think having a grasp on the dynamics of eating and some of the evidence really allows optimization of any gym or even life goal. Nutrition is simple yet complicated and is a big part of daily life, understanding it really takes some pressure off of the process.

In this text there is science communicated via citations. It is important to understand that all research reports means, or the averages, of the results. That means that these concepts should be taken as a general construct to assist in your journey, as some results are higher than the reported average and some are lower. This is not the only downfall to research. There are many limitations, and there is no such thing as a perfect study, especially when humans are the subjects. We humans have a life to live and can't be studied in an isolated environment the way some other species and cells can. Understand that the results of research provides information that is applicable to your life, and being able to use it to your advantage is the most important thing to take away. It should not be viewed as law.

I hope you enjoy Part I of the four part series of *Healthy Body, Healthy Mind, Healthy Life.*

-Joe Boone

1 WELLNESS, THE CENTER OF PROGRESSION

HEALTH, FITNESS, AND WELLNESS DEFINED

Health may be defined as the absence of disease or a diseased state. According to this definition, when you hear someone say they want to become "healthier," they are, in a sense, admitting their current lifestyle decisions are not optimal. Whether it is eating processed food, fast food, excess food, getting too little exercise, or other harmful behaviors, these actions keep us from living a healthy lifestyle [1 – 3]. This is health as it is related to the physical body.

The term "health" may be further broken down into subcomponents, including mental and social aspects. Being healthy is not just the absence of disease in the body. It is also the well-being of the mind and an individual's psychosocial life, or the relationships a person has with other people. These three things are tightly woven together, and this chapter will bring some light to how integral their relationship is.

There is a fourth aspect to a person's health that goes deeper than what the eye can see, and that is spiritual health. The physical, mental, and social subcomponents are manifestations of the physical health of the body and its parts. The mind is made up of physical organs and social relationships are made of people, and all of these things are tangible parts of life. Unlike these aspects of health, the spiritual component is not as easy to see, but it's equally important. Spirituality and spiritual health generally mean having a sense of meaning or purpose and a connection to a set of values which guide that purpose. How you establish spiritual health and your spirituality is dependent on your belief systems.

Spirituality has a big impact on your life. Are you able to understand the meaning of the things that happen? Are you able to accept there are things you cannot change? Your spiritualty has a huge impact on your mental health. If your perception does not allow you to accept what is happening around you, then your mindset is altered, and that is what determines your mental and ultimately even your emotional health.

Fitness can be defined as a measurable level of ability. Generally, in biology, an organism's fitness level is judged by whether or not it can reproduce and survive its environment [4]. Is the organism fit enough to pass on its genetic material? The popular slogan "survival of the fittest" says it all. In physical fitness this translates to many things one being reduction of disease risk, which allows a person to live a longer and healthier life. For example, level of fitness has a direct relationship to risk of early death [5], the more fit the less likely to die early. That results in the ability of a fit person to live a longer and potentially more enjoyable life than someone who is less fit.

Wellness is defined as a general sense of well-being. Simply, it is the compilation of health and fitness-- the absence of disease, a highly functioning mind, relationships that are mutually beneficial, and in a general sense a high level of functioning in your body and across life. Are there some limitations to that? Yes, but we can all strive to improve our individual levels by first understanding what they mean.

HOW THEY ARE RELATED

Defining and differentiating between health, fitness, and wellness helps us understand how they are all different. But it also helps us understand how they are linked to each other. Let's take a look at their relationship. Do you specifically know how your level of health is tied to your fitness and wellness?

Under all three terms there are many components. These include emotional, mental, relational, social, muscular, cardiovascular, and financial. The list could go on, but the fact is that the components of health, fitness, and wellness all come together and shape how you live your life.

The healthier you are the greater potential you have to function at a higher output in the tangible and intangible portions of your life. It may be variable from person to person, but overall the more fit you are physically, mentally, socially, and spiritually, the greater potential there is for improved quality of wellness across life as a spectrum. Health manifests in so many other ways that influence your quality of life, which is why health and wealth have a relationship. Health often correlates with fitness [5], and therefore wellness. The more well you are the greater your potential to excel in other areas of your life. Is wealth necessarily tied to the amount of zeros in your bank account? No, there is much more to wealth.

Wealth is subjective to what your goals in life are, and it is up to you to decide what makes you wealthy. Is it having a large family with people that support and love each other? Is it accomplishing personal career goals? Is it having a small group of friends to call on when you need them the most? Is it being educated? Is it financial wealth? This is something you must decide for yourself. The work you have to do to reach those goals will depend on your overall health and fitness.

The likelihood of you being able to perform at the top of your game and be wealthy is not high if your body is burdened with disease. Success is not likely if you're on the lower echelons of physical capability, or your general sense of being is negative. How can you have a high output on pursing a goal if your emotional state is out of whack? How can you achieve a wealthy life, whatever that means to you, if you look at the world in a negative light? How can you achieve what you want to achieve without generally being well?

It is not impossible, but the more healthy you are, the more fit you are likely to be and the more likely you are to have a higher sense of well-being. This manifests all across your life.

Understanding how to get there is a very dynamic and ever-changing path, so it is important to understand that the psychological aspect may be the hardest part. Can you use that mind of yours to evaluate what needs to be evaluated and accept what needs to be accepted? Motivation, psychology and mindset are highly intertwined and have a relationship comparable to that of the molecules that make up our cells. Your ability to develop your mindset and know that there will be failures is crucial; you have to be able to pick yourself up and learn from every experience. After all, failure is just another word for lesson. The people that you view as successful did not make it to the place they are in life without stumbling down the path and being beaten up by its obstacles. They took the beating, got back up, and continued on stronger.

Obviously, health and wellness are linked together. But to reach our goals and fully understand each aspect, we must break it down into the specific components. In *Healthy Body, Healthy Mind, Healthy Life Part I: Nutrition* we look at the many aspects of the diet in an attempt to realize the importance of nutrition on the path to wellness.

NUTRITION

One of the most crucial portions of achieving all around wellness happens to be what you put into your body. Everyone has heard the phrase "you are what you eat." At some level everything you put in your body is processed, used, stored, or excreted. What you put in your body is broken down and digested; after that the remnants are used to build new cells, make energy for those cells, and become part of the many processes that your body conducts every second of every day. You are what you eat. What you eat is the foundation of your cellular development.

The definition of nutrition, when applied to the body, is the science of the compounds that make up food and how those compounds influence and nourish the human body [6]. These compounds are broken down into six classes: carbohydrates, fats, proteins, vitamins, minerals, and water. Carbohydrates, fats, and proteins are needed in larger quantities and are therefore known as the macronutrients. Vitamins and minerals are needed in smaller quantities and consequently are known as micronutrients. The final and most significant nutrient is water. The second biggest difference between the macronutrients and the other nutrients is that macronutrients supply energy through kilocalories while the others do not.

Good nutrition plays a role in lowering the risk and reducing the severity of many chronic diseases. In fact, it has been called the best medicine you can take. At the same time poor nutrition does seem to have a relationship with poor health [7]. Armed with the proper knowledge of nutrition, *you* can improve your health as well as allow for many more benefits. Remember this statement as your knowledge base on nutrition grows.

2 AN INTRODUCTION TO MACRONUTRIENTS

The macronutrients provide energy in the form of kilocalories, or what are more commonly known as calories. They provide these calories in different amounts and play crucial roles in the body's daily processes. Because of these roles there have been standard recommendations made for intake of these nutrients. The Acceptable Macronutrient Distribution Range (AMDR) states that carbohydrates should compose forty-five to sixty-five percent of total daily caloric intake, fats should compose twenty to thirty-five percent, and protein should compose ten to thirty-five percent [8]. However, these are loose guidelines – the distribution an individual requires is based on his or her individual characteristics.

Fats provide nine calories per gram, while carbohydrates and proteins provide four calories per gram. The bottom line is that fats are more energy dense per gram than the other macronutrients, but that is not the reason the body requires a different amount of fat in comparison to the other two. The reasons they are required in different amounts are rooted in the other roles the nutrients play inside the body.

Fats, in a general sense, are used when the body is exerting minimal or lower levels of effort. They go through aerobic metabolism and provide a lot of energy per molecule. Carbohydrates are used at higher levels of exertion during anaerobic energy production. They are used where the energy demand is high and the duration is short. Although protein provides calories just like the other macronutrients, it is important to know that protein is not generally relied on for its energy-providing ability. In normal conditions the body has many functions outside of energy which protein is used for, and this is primarily why the guidelines for protein intake are set lower than fat and carbohydrate.

Proteins are generally only used as an energy source when they are absolutely needed. In fact, even in prolonged exercise where other fuel sources are depleted, proteins only contribute up to ten percent of the total energy expenditure output. The significance of proteins being used for energy is that their main role lies in other functions including tissue growth, repair, and maintenance, immune system function, whole body maintenance, biological transport of nutrients, hormone function, and others. The body requires certain amounts of protein every day to perform these regular functions. When the body is forced to use proteins for energy, they don't necessarily come from foods you have eaten. Instead they may come from tissues inside your body, like skeletal muscle.

There are two general energy pathways where the macronutrients are catabolized, or broken down, and energy is produced -- aerobic and anaerobic. We can look at the energy systems that break down fats, carbohydrates, and proteins like faucets. The faucets function for the different macronutrients, so imagine there is a faucet for each one. In this example, the faucet for fats is constantly dripping. The fat molecule has to go through a process that is a little more complex than that of carbohydrates, but provides a larger amount of energy, and is therefore used under low levels of exertion. When comparing fats to carbohydrates, carbohydrates are more easily converted into energy and used during higher levels of exertion.

There are two types of fats: saturated and unsaturated. Generally speaking, saturated fats are found in animal foods and unsaturated fats are found in plants and oils. The saturated fats are deemed the unhealthier of the two. They have a more rigid structure and higher melting point, which means that once inside the human body they may be more likely to stick to surfaces and create build up. Their structure is due to the hydrogen-bonding in the saturated fat molecule. The carbon atoms in fat molecules hold bonds with hydrogen atoms, and in saturated fats all of the possible bonds are made, creating a molecule that cannot be bonded with any more hydrogens. This is why it is known as being saturated, as it is saturated with hydrogens. The unsaturated fat does not have as many hydrogens bonded to it and is therefore a less rigid molecule that has a lower melting point. This is why unsaturated fats are oils at room temperature and saturated fats are solid in the same conditions.

Outside of the two naturally found fats there are also man-made fats. These are known as hydrogenated oils, or trans-fats. Hydrogenated oils are created when extra hydrogen atoms are added to unsaturated fats to change the molecule from an oil to a solid. This conversion from unsaturated to saturated gives the fat and the product it is in a longer shelf life. It also allows the package to show it does not have any saturated fats in it, when on a molecular level it actually does. These are found in processed food products.

Fats are a very efficient source of energy, and seeing they provide a larger energy yield shows this. During day-to-day activities like desk work, walking, eating, and driving, fats are the main source of energy.

Energy utilization with the faucets for carbohydrates and fats are related. As exertion level increases, the ratio of fat utilization to carbohydrate utilization changes to favor carbohydrates [9]. Simply put, the higher the exertion level, the more carbohydrate is used, and the lower the exertion the more fat is used. The concept of the energy faucet is crucial to understanding how calories are burned.

A common phrase that comes up in relation to this topic is the fat burning zone. At a certain point in intensity the utilization of fat is at its highest, and a heart rate and training intensity can be associated with that point [10]. Keep in mind there is more to be considered, since we have learned the faucets have relationships and all macronutrients can be used for energy.

The three macronutrients are broken down into smaller molecules that we can consider their building blocks. Carbohydrates are made of sugars or saccharides, proteins are made of amino acids, and fats of fatty acids. They do have other components, but the saccharide, amino acid, and fatty acid are the most significant of their composition in energy yield and metabolism.

SUGARS

Carbohydrates are composed of sugars, or more precisely saccharides. The many types of saccharides are all made of the same elements; carbon, oxygen, and hydrogen. This is where the name carb-o-hydrate comes from. The source will determine how many of each atom are present in the sugar molecule. The body uses glucose as its blood sugar, and most of the sugar that is ingested is transformed into glucose. Glucose is also what plants and animals store carbohydrates as in their cells. Glucoses' chemical formula is 6 carbons, 12 hydrogens, and 6 oxygens. All sugars are in this 1:2:1 proportion.

Sugars are easily identified on nutrition labels, as most of them end in *ose*, as in glucose, sucrose, maltose, fructose, dextrose, and galactose, for example. These each represent a different form of sugar. The important takeaway is that sugars fall under the class of carbohydrates. As a food source a carbohydrate food can provide many benefits and other nutrients, even if there is sugar in it.

Amino Acids

Proteins are composed of substances called amino acids. In total there are twenty of them, nine of which must be consumed through food. These are known as essential amino acids. The other eleven can be created from substances within the adult body and are known as non-essential amino acids.

When it comes to food sources of the essential amino acids (EAAs) a food that contains all nine is known as a complete protein, and one that does not is known as an incomplete protein. This is the major difference between protein found in animal and plant sources, animal sources are complete and most plant sources are incomplete. This is one of the main concerns for those that prescribe to a plant-based diet. As protein is very important in the processes of the human body, consuming enough of the EAAs is crucial.

The most significant amino acid is Leucine, due to its direct role in upregulating (or turning on) the cellular protein synthesis pathway mTOR, which allows cells to build new proteins [11-13]. Meats are the best source of complete proteins, but you can eat different types of foods that contain the different EAAs to satisfy this need. When this is done correctly, the protein sources complement each other in their amino acid composition and can satisfy the body's requirement.

These twenty amino acids can be put into many combinations to make many proteins. These many proteins include our muscle fibers (skeletal, cardiac, and smooth), enzymes, hormones, and many other biological substances. Proteins are very specific, and their shape gives them their function. The functions they perform range from enzymatic action, structure rigidity (from soft tissue to bone), immunity, biochemical molecule transporters, connective tissue and contractile fiber components, and many others. Due to proteins' many functions in the body and the body's protein turnover where whole-body protein is constantly being replaced [14], a significant amount of protein is needed in the diet. In fact, it has been found that meeting protein requirements is more important than meeting energy needs especially in pathological or stressed states [15]. Coupling this with findings that show amino acid intake, specifically Leucine, positively influences hunger control and satiety [16], all comes together with implications for just how important dietary protein is.

FATTY ACIDS

The fatty acids are the tails of the fat molecule. They are attached to the head of the molecule, a glycerol. The term triglyceride refers to how each fat molecule has three fatty acids and one glycerol. When our body is ready to use dietary fats for energy, the fatty acids are split from the glycerol and those fatty acids are broken down into their individual pieces.

Because of the make-up of the different fatty acids, those that are saturated are more solid at room temperature. Most significantly, they may have a greater impact on cholesterol levels in the blood in comparison to unsaturated fats [17]. In a general sense, high-fat meals cause conditions for greater plaque accumulation and increase atherosclerotic potential in the body's vessels [18]. However, fat intake does have its purposes, like vitamin and mineral content, endocrine health, lubrication, and providing biological building blocks [19], just to list a few.

There is not actually a Recommended Daily Allowance (RDA) set for fat intake, but if we use the AMDR as an example we can see a manifestation of how dietary fat has its purposes and benefits. Recalling the importance of amino acid and protein intake, fatty acids and fats are comparable in importance because of the roles the fat molecule and its components play in the body. For one, the body uses fatty acids for energy, which is crucial since we are made of trillions of cells that are constantly needing new energy. Secondly, the body breaks down fatty acids and can transform them into different components that are used for other functions such as biological transporters and building blocks. Those include nutrient storage and transport, hormones, new and damaged cell components, thermoregulation, bone deposition, and others.

In comparing the different building blocks of the macronutrients, we can see that they all provide benefits. But there are other things that must be considered, such as the source and the application of the energy. Depending on your goals, health status, and many other factors, macronutrient manipulations can go many ways. In order to be able to properly understand nutrition you must first know why it would be beneficial or not beneficial to make a decision about the individual macronutrient.

The exact distributions of each are highly disputed, but what cannot be disputed is that they all have functions in the body and their applications can vary from person to person.

3 METABOLISM AND ENERGY BALANCE

Understanding nutrition at a lower level is important, and now that we have gone over the building blocks of those components it is time to use them as an aid in looking at the bigger picture of nutrition. The words metabolism and diet, food labels and food product marketing are highly intertwined in our daily lives. Understanding these things and the many others laid out in this text will help you build your base on nutritional knowledge.

The recommended daily calorie allowance for most adults is 2,000 calories. This number has created a fixation in Americans on calories and counting how many are consumed at each meal, which takes the emphasis off of the nutrients. When you focus on calories instead of nutrients you run the risk of limiting certain foods and not allowing your body the full range of nutrients needed for maximum function.

Also, that number is very general. In fact, the literature that sets the 2,000 calorie Recommended Daily Allowance (RDA) also recognizes a variance of about 1,000 calories per day between adult females and males respectively [20]. On top of that, the RDA has a role in label standardization. The 2,000 calorie diet was created to provide a standard so food labels could display Daily Value (DV) percentages, allowing a standard for comparison purposes. This was done to give the consumer an idea of what they were getting out of the food. While the standard has its purpose, the human factor means every person's caloric requirement is different. That said, 2,000 calories per day may be accurate for one person but could be completely wrong for another.

The word metabolism is thrown around very commonly. From the conversations between friends about how you wish you had someone else's to the fad work outs that claim to boost it. But most people don't know the real definition. Metabolism is the total number of processes that occur across your entire body, including the ones that "burn" calories and those that do not. This means it spans the entire body across its trillions of cells. That includes all processes, from making new cells in the skeleton to the molecular processes your lungs perform to the processes your arteries and veins perform to keep blood flowing to the right places.

A person's metabolism is taken into account when determining their daily energy requirement. Each individual's caloric requirement and metabolism is varied based upon activity level, age, biological sex, height, and total body mass (weight). There are other factors like weight or fitness goals, health status, and genetics, that are less cut and dried. For example, genetic testing could tell you how you metabolize certain nutrients, but a test like that is not readily available and can be expensive.

Different types of people require significantly different numbers of daily calories. For example; large athletes can require 10,000 or more; recreational exercisers can require between 2,500 and 5,000; runners can require around 4,000, and all around healthy and active individuals may require as much as 3,000. But without knowing the individual's specific characteristics, those numbers are shots in the dark.

There are three things that come together to compile someone's total caloric output for a given day. The first is Resting Metabolic Rate (RMR), which is the most influential of the three, providing 60-75 percent of total energy expenditure [21]. RMR, which is simply the amount of energy your body requires to run its systems, can be determined through a couple of different formulas. The two classic formulas are the Harris Benedict and the Mifflin Jeor, and there are also formulas created by the World Health Organization (WHO), the Food and Agriculture Organization (FAO), and the United Nations University (UNU). All of these formulas provide a general approximation [22]. The most accurate way to measure RMR and metabolic rate is through direct calorimetry. Unfortunately this is not a very accessible test, but if you do have access it is the best way to determine your energy needs.

Activity level is the second of the three influencers on an individual's metabolism. Activity level can make up as much as 30 percent of a person's metabolism [21], however the percentage at which activity level influences metabolic rate is variable and can range from day to day and person to person. Physical activity can be factored into the different formulas by multiplying the RMR by an activity factor (1.0 – 1.7).

The third and final portion of total metabolic rate is the Thermal Effect of Feeding (TEF). TEF is the amount of energy or heat used and/or created during the digestion of food. TEF accounts for approximately 10 percent of energy output [21], but again the number is variable based on the person and other influencing factors. One of those variables is the type of food ingested. Generally, protein foods have the highest TEF, but the size of the meal has been found to be most influential [23]. The best way to interpret this is that eating fewer meals that are larger instead of eating many meals that are smaller may provide a way to increase caloric output via digesting food. The main thing to take away from TEF is that it takes energy to digest food; protein foods are most influential of the macronutrients on TEF and the larger the meal the more energy it takes to digest.

Now that we see the dynamics of individual metabolism, we can look at fat loss a little more in depth. Each pound of body fat contains about 3,500 calories of energy. In order to lose just one pound of body fat, a 3,500 calorie energy deficit is required. This number allows us to understand why fat loss is so difficult. Understanding what makes up total energy expenditure provides a foundation for how manipulating dietary intake can make the goal more attainable.

Creating an energy deficit requires energy intake to be less than energy output. Creating a deficit forces your body to resort to stored energy for its needs.

On the opposite side, if you are trying to gain weight then you must create an energy surplus. When you are creating an energy surplus fat gain can be expected. Our bodies only store limited amounts of carbohydrate and amino acids. No matter the nutrients consumed, if the calories are over the requirement there will be some fat storage. With the appropriate program for your goals you can increase muscle mass and even carbohydrate storage, but because of limited storage for those you should expect some fat gain.

To eat for optimal conditions you have to give your body what it needs in the right amounts and limit or exclude the things that it doesn't. To achieve these things here are some general guidelines: eat the appropriate portions according to your energy needs, limit or exclude processed and fried foods, and eat enough protein and fiber.

The body is constantly making new energy. This can either be from newly ingested food or stores within the body of carbohydrate, protein, and fat. This is an important concept to understand when it comes to the goals of your nutrition. It means that the body is always metabolizing something, even if you haven't recently eaten. Knowing this is essential to understanding when it is best for you to eat. The reaction that occurs immediately upon the body recognizing calories, and to a more pronounced effect carbohydrate, is that it tells the pancreas to release insulin. Insulin then acts to reduce the sugar in the blood by telling the cells to take it in. But in doing this, insulin inhibits the mechanisms that facilitate fat metabolism. This is something that has to be taken into consideration, especially when the goal is fat loss. If you are always snacking on sugary foods, then your fat metabolism is being greatly reduced. However, for some it is beneficial to eat carbohydrate more frequently because insulin and other associated hormones have an indirect anabolic effect on muscle protein synthesis and balance [24, 25]. Eating the appropriate portions according to your energy needs when you need to eat them, limiting or excluding processed and fried foods, and eating enough protein and fiber are all crucial to maintaining health in the body.

In our busy society, one of the most difficult parts of maintaining good nutrition is staying away from processed foods. When possible you should always opt for the real food option. Many food-like products have replaced the real foods that we as humans are meant to digest. The convenience and cost of processed foods are the major factors that play into nutrient source selection.

Other factors that influence a person's selection are taste, culture, social interaction, environment, habits, genetics, stress, and emotions [26 - 29]. Knowing these things gives you a better understanding as to why you may choose the foods you do.

Paying attention to macronutrients is the simplest way to follow your overall nutrition. We use the word follow because when it comes to nutritional intake, tracking your every calorie becomes very difficult. Not only that, but I find people become fixed on a number that will fluctuate from day-to-day. What is more important than calories is the nutrient density of the food and establishing good behaviors surrounding food. Basically, you should pick foods for the nutrients they contain instead of what the label says are in it and eating should be part of the big picture. The foods that have the most nutrients tend to be those that do not require a label. Processing procedures damage the naturally occurring nutrients in foods. Remember there are six nutrient classes: carbohydrate, fat, protein, vitamins, minerals, and water. They are all significant.

Changing dietary habits can be stressful and very difficult. If you make yourself count every calorie you are only adding more stress to that process. When that stress becomes too great it will push you in the opposite direction, back to old habits. When a rebound like this happens because of the stress of a new clean eating plan it can cause worse eating behaviors than before the change was made. Setting yourself up for success in a nutritional program means making the change manageable. Eat things that you like and begin to experiment with things that you think you may like. Make it a process that continues to evolve and is fun. If you get to a place where you have specific goals, calorie counting can be a way to accomplish those, but that does not mean everyone needs to count every calorie.

Now that you understand calorie and nutrient intake and its relation to energy output, it's time to take a look at some more specific components of nutrition.

4 CARBOHYDRATES

Carbohydrates are found in grains, vegetables, fruits, beans, and legumes. In fact, carbohydrates are found in practically all foods, but what determines whether a food gets classified as a carbohydrate is the concentration of carbohydrate in the food. This same classification applies to all food types, so if a food is mostly protein it will be a protein food, if it is mostly fat it will be a fat food, even though they may contain amounts of the other macronutrients.

Carbohydrates, or carbs, as they are commonly called, are an important macronutrient in the context of energy supply. Carbohydrates are stored predominantly in the liver and muscle cells. They circulate the body's fluids as some cells use them exclusively for energy (i.e. red blood cells). It was once thought that carbohydrates were the only fuel some neural cells would use, but as nutrition and physiological science has evolved, we have learned more about our body's ability to fuel itself. There are trillions of cells all using energy by metabolizing the pieces of macronutrients. Interestingly, the body can make its own glucose out of other compounds through a process called gluconeogenesis. All of this is very significant information, but there is much to be considered outside of the food, like exercise.

Carbohydrates are like any macro and should be consumed in moderation. Many chronic conditions have been linked to metabolic issues with dysregulated *cellular* carbohydrate metabolism, including cancers, inflammatory conditions of the gut, and neuro and muscular degeneration [30 – 35]. Carbs seem to have earned a negative cloud of attention. Apparently if you eat them you will add body fat to your frame; in reality it's not the food that makes you fat but your behaviors that surround food and exercise. Any nutrient that contains calories will make you fat if you eat too much of it and don't use the energy it gives you.

Grains and bread are the most common examples of carbohydrates, but they are not the only source. Recall carbohydrates are sugar molecules that are joined together. They are what plants and animals use to store energy. With that in mind, we can see how bread and grains are not the only way to get them. Other sources include but are not limited to fruit, vegetables, legumes, and beans.

Processing is one of the biggest factors to consider in carbohydrate food selection. Enrichment and refinement are two common processes performed to lengthen the shelf-life of grain products, but they also have other effects. In refinement, nutrients are removed to facilitate lengthening of the shelf-life. The nutrients that are lost include the fiber, fat, phytochemicals (plant specific chemicals), vitamins, and minerals in the foods. This essentially leaves sugar and the protein in the grain. Since wheat is the most common we will examine it. It is a whole grain before it is refined and is comprised of three parts – the bran, germ, and endosperm. Refinement is a process where these parts are separated and some of the nutrients, like the fat, are removed. This is the reason refined grains appear more white and have a longer shelf life. Enrichment is a process where some of nutrients are added back, but only a fraction are and important nutrients like fiber are not.

Another significant consideration in carbohydrate foods is the Glycemic Index (GI). Many people consider the GI as a way to rate whether or not a carbohydrate food is healthy or unhealthy. This is a common misconception. To understand why that is the case we must first understand how exactly a food is rated on the GI and why it is rated that way. The prefix gly- refers to sugar, so we automatically know that the GI has something to do with sugar content in the food. What it is actually measuring is the impact the food has on blood sugar and the time associated with the impact. The higher the GI rating of a food the more dramatic of an impact on blood sugar and the faster and longer that rise in blood sugar occurs and lasts.

It is not actually the sugar content of the food that determines the GI, it is the insulin response the body has to the specific food. In fact, the sugars in both low and high glycemic foods go through digestion and enter the blood at about the same rate. The difference is that there is a more dramatic insulin reaction from low GI foods to properly regulate the new blood sugar and clear it out via cellular uptake [36-39]. This is important because high blood sugar can cause damage. Consider the damage that occurs with chronic hyperglycemia in diabetics, sugar is sticky inside the body just like it is on the outside.

This is not to say that high GI foods are bad for you, as many fruits have high GI ratings and contain many essential nutrients. Ingesting a food high on the GI can be used to provide the working muscle with sugar as a fuel without worrying about insulin signaling.

When selecting a carbohydrate food it is appropriate to consider the GI, the nutrient density, and proximity of ingestion to exercise, because outside of insulin exercise is the only other major signal for the cells to take in blood sugar.

If you are choosing between carbohydrate foods in the perspective of health the main things to consider are nutrient density and processing. The GI rating can be used, but it should not be a staple reference. Do not forget that processing removes nutrients. One of the major nutrients that is removed is the fiber. With fiber being so important and lacking in most diets, this should be a great indicator on which foods to stay away from. Ultimately the less processing the food goes through before it gets to you the better.

FIBER

Fiber is a carbohydrate. Even though it falls under the macronutrient of carbohydrate, it is listed separately on food labels and spoken about as if it has different functions. So, what could the reasoning behind that be?

The human body uses enzymes to break down food. In order to do that the enzymes break chemical bonds in between the linked molecules. However, the human body does not produce all of the enzymes necessary to completely break down fiber molecules. The majority of the digestion of fiber comes from the mashing and tearing of the teeth and sloshing of the stomach, and there are still relatively large pieces left in the digestive system once it continues past the stomach. When it reaches the large intestines it has a different role in comparison to other foods. Large pieces move through the intestines and slide through in a foam-like manner, picking up the leftovers of poor digestion [40]. Fiber flushes this waste out of the body. This is one of the reasons why fiber is important even if we do not fully digest it. And you will find if your diet is low in fiber and out of nowhere you eat a food that is high in fiber it can prompt a bowel movement much sooner than you normally would expect. Fiber also plays a significant role in feeding the micro-biome.

There are two concerns with low fiber intake and the large intestines. Waste accumulation in the large intestines has been associated with colon cancer. This is because waste is toxic, and when not flushed out properly that toxic material is sitting stagnant on top of intestinal cells for extended periods of time. The other concern is a condition called diverticulosis [41]. This is when an accumulation of waste has occupied an area for so long that it becomes a pouch, or a diverticula. If that happens it is dangerous because the pouch can break and release toxic waste into the rest of the body. Think about it like a plastic grocery bag you put too many things in and the plastic stretched. Once formed, the pouches cannot heal and return to their original state as flat areas in the large intestines. These conditions can be prevented with proper fiber intake [42]. Most adults get about 15 grams per day. That is very low in comparison to the recommended daily amount of 25 grams for women and 38 grams for men [20]. Research shows adequate fiber reduces risk of these conditions [42 – 44]. Research suggests that adequate fiber intake can assist in the reduction of glycemic and insulin impact of foods, decrease plasma cholesterol and lipids, decrease fat storage, improve insulin sensitivity, and improvement in feelings of fullness [45]. Specifically for cholesterol-based molecules in the intestines, fiber is able to attach and help the body pass it before it is absorbed into the blood. Put simply, fiber is an essential nutrient that has a long list of benefits that includes overall health and is very influential in nutrient absorption.

5 FATS

Fats are found in more foods than they are thought to be. In fact, they are found in almost every food, including plants. Each fat molecule can contain both unsaturated and saturated fatty acids, which means that, generally speaking, all fats could be composed of both types. This is the same concept as the majority macronutrient concentration determining a food's classification. For example, beans are generally considered a high protein food, but because their majority make up is carbohydrate they are technically a carbohydrate. This concept is applicable on the classification of a fat or triglyceride. If a triglyceride has two fatty acids that are saturated and one that is unsaturated, then it will be considered saturated. Conversely, if it has two that are unsaturated and one that is saturated then in will be unsaturated. We can see that fat content is more complex than the nutrition label lets on.

The significance of fat in energy is that it is generally used in low-level exertion, but there are many other considerations to be accounted for. The two main locations for body storage of fat are subcutaneous and visceral. Subcutaneous fat is the fat that is stored just beneath the skin, and visceral fat is stored in the viscera, the area that contains the abdominal organs. Between the two sexes, men are more likely to store fat in the viscera, while women are more likely to store it subcutaneously. Visceral fat is where the term beer belly comes from. It is characterized with the distention and hardening of the abdominal area. The fat is stored on and around the abdominal organs, like the liver, and can push the abdominal wall out. Visceral fat is very dangerous due to the proximity to the vital organs, but primarily because its impact on the liver and metabolism [46, 47].

The vitals or vital organs are commonly heard terms in the context of health care. A vital organ is one that is required to maintain life. Obviously the heart and lungs fall into that category, but with the storage of fat in the abdomen the one that is most significantly impacted is the liver. The liver has many roles in maintaining life. Those roles include processing oxygen-rich blood, processing venous blood, producing bile, regulating cholesterol, and processing toxins. In its processing of the arterial and venous blood the liver has other functions as well, which are all tied to metabolism and blood constituent regulation.

When food is ingested it goes through the digestive tract, and once it reaches the small intestines absorption begins. When nutrients are absorbed they go into the venous blood, and the first place they reach is the liver. This is why the association of poor liver health is tied to excessive alcohol consumption. One of the things the liver does is filter the toxins that come through. With that, all nutrients that are absorbed reach the liver for processing. The liver acts as somewhat of the nutrient door man and regulates what nutrients are stored, put into circulation, or transformed into other molecules. That includes the control of blood sugar, amino acid, cholesterol, and triglyceride levels. With excess fat storage around the organ that controls these things comes the impairment of its functioning. For this reason, visceral fat has a relationship with increased risk in developing metabolic conditions such as Type-II Diabetes [48].

On top of that, visceral fat is much more difficult to get rid of than other fat. Knowing this is important to the psychological portion of a fat loss goal. If you are going to be fighting a hard battle you must prepare yourself, you must know your enemy. But, you must also know the tools you have at your disposal and how to use them.

The recommendations for fat were once built upon nutritional science that spoke to the negative impacts of its intake. However, this is an area of nutritional research that is currently receiving a lot of attention. Research on fat in the diet suggests that the intake of higher amounts increases the body's ability to utilize fat as fuel [49, 50], and it may provide other benefits that require more research. Since the body is capable of storing an unlimited amount of energy as fat, this provides interesting implications. It does not mean that fats should be coming from fried foods, trans-fats, or other fats found in processed foods. What it does mean is that fat intake should not be limited to the extreme that some like to promote. What should also be considered is the research application of the ketogenic diet in fat loss, metabolic heath, and clinical populations. The research indicates that this high-fat diet has impacts and results that include anti-convulsant properties in epileptic patients, is therapeutic toward types of cancer, fosters weight-loss, and brain health [49 – 55], however just because there is some research to show that it could provide these effects does not mean everyone should be using keto.

With all of these considerations on fat, we can see its importance in normal physiology. Dietary fat has roles in nutrient storage and transport, hormones, building new and repairing damaged cells, thermoregulation, bone mineral deposition, energy balance, and other functions. The name fat automatically has a negative connotation that is not conducive to the potentially positive impacts it has biologically. It is important to understand that it is required in the diet, but the specific application is dependent on individual factors like health and goals.

6 PROTEINS

Proteins are found in meat, poultry, fish, plant sources, and anything with amino acids. When considering protein, most people think of meat sources, but there are many other places to get protein and amino acids. Did you know that rice and peas are considered a good source of protein? Did you know that if you eat rice and beans together, or even in the same day, it satisfies the requirement for a complete protein?

The problem with looking to get your protein intake from mostly meat used to be the high content of fat that was also in meats. However, not all meat is high in fat. On top of that, research suggests that fat may not be the cause of the problems we used to associate with it, and some research is even beginning to show that high-fat diets and the byproducts of fat metabolism can be beneficial, depending on the application [56, 57]. In a large study, researchers found that compared to vegetarians, non-vegetarians (non-meat restricted) had a greater risk of dying from ischemic heart attack [58]. But one year later the same team of researchers published there were no significant differences between the vegetarians and non-vegetarians in mortality from cerebrovascular disease, stomach cancer, colorectal cancer, lung cancer, breast cancer, prostate cancer, or all other causes combined [59]. That leads to the question of whether it is really the meat that is causing the issues, or is there some other factor or set of factors playing into this?

Most of the studies in the past that showed it was the meat eater that had worse health than the vegetarian did not control for other variables, most significantly lifestyle. A 2015 study looked at individuals with Non-Alcoholic Fatty Liver Disease (NAFLD), a condition that is commonly associated with metabolic disorders and consequently poor nutrition and inactivity. This study found that the risk factors associated with NAFLD are sedentary lifestyle and family history of metabolic syndrome, as well as consumption of meat/fish, spicy foods, fried foods, and tea [60]. The most important of the variables is listed first, lifestyle, and this shows us that it is not meat alone that impacts metabolic health and disease risk. An additional study performed on a group of over 250,000 people in 2017 found there is no evidence that following a vegetarian diet provides protection against all-cause mortality in comparison to eating meat [61], again showing the importance of things outside of meat intake.

The other major consideration of protein intake is independent of the source. Nitrogen, which is a part of proteins and amino acids, is released during digestion. A common school of thought surrounds protein intake with a negative impact of high nitrogen on the body. Nitrogen dysregulation is related to kidney failure. The term protein toxicity is tied to the idea that a diet is too high in protein. It was once thought that high protein intake negatively impacted kidney health via high levels of nitrogen. The RDA sets nitrogen intake at 105 mg per kilogram of bodyweight per day. That requirement is set based on the nitrogen balance where the body rids itself of nitrogen from protein turnover in urine, sweat, and feces every day [20]. Nitrogen balance, and ingesting enough to replace what is lost, is important in maintaining healthy, metabolically active muscle tissue along with the many other proteins. In fact, there is evidence that suggests the RDA may be too low to provide positive nitrogen balance and replenish what is lost through your body's normal function [62].

What this tells us is that if you use the RDA, you may not be getting enough nitrogen in your diet, let alone be ingesting an amount that has any potential to damage to your kidneys. It has also been found that long-term, low-protein intake via plant-based diets has the same effect on kidney function as a non-restricted diet that includes meat [63]. All of this tells us that protein intake is not as damaging as some will express, and that the idea of increasing the protein content of a diet may be warranted, but it is always dependent on the situation.

It is my opinion that one of the major variables that is not considered in the research stating that meat-eaters are at higher risk for disease development is that the typical meat eater prescribes to all-around unhealthy eating habits (and lack of activity) including high intake of processed foods. We can consider that there is a potential for the intake of processed foods and low levels of physical activity to impact results of studies that do not control the other parts of participant's diet when looking at protein and meat.

When we look at meat and protein intake we need to look at both sides of the issue. Are there risks to a high intake of protein and meat? Yes, there potentially are, but there are risks to overconsuming anything, and it is becoming evident that the risk of excessive protein intake may not be as high as is publicly communicated. What is interesting about increasing protein intake is that there seems to be more benefits than risks. In fact, increasing protein intake has been linked to better control of hormones that regulate hunger. In one study, researchers specifically found that increasing protein intake while reducing total caloric intake had the effect of increasing the feeling of fullness and satiety [64]. And recall, protein foods have the biggest impact on TEF and increasing metabolic rate.

Fiber intake is crucial in all nutritional applications, but in regards to meat intake fiber may be even more important. The availability of processed meats can make them the easier choice in comparison to a healthier alternative. We briefly covered some processing procedures for carbohydrates, and that the goal of processing is to create a product that has a longer shelf life and greater return on investment for the producer. That said, the nutrient content of the food is not the same as it would be unprocessed, as some things are added and some things are removed. Are there potential benefits to food processing? Yes. Some of those include fortifying a product with micronutrients like vitamins and minerals, but those are not the only things that are done to the food. What should not be ignored is that the source and preparation of meat is significant in its impact on the body.

Considering what fiber does for digestion it becomes extremely important when meat is eaten, especially if that meat is processed.

One of the benefits of eating plant-based proteins is that they contain phytochemicals and fiber. Phytochemicals are exclusively found in plants. One benefit to plant-based proteins is that they are much leaner and contain minimal saturated fats. But as you've seen in our talking about nutrition, it is better to balance than to limit your intake. Plant-based proteins have benefits, but so do animal foods, which contain zoochemicals. They both have their own benefits to nourishing the human body.

Another comparison of animal versus plant is their exclusive nutrients. There are certain nutrients that are only found in meats and not in plants. Vitamin B12, Vitamin D, creatine, magnesium, and phosphorous are just a few examples of nutrients that are difficult to get into a vegetarian diet. Fruits, vegetables, beans, legumes, and whole grains all have great nutrient density and provide their own benefits. That said, variety in dietary intake allows for a great variance of nutrient supply, and we can see how restriction of a food type may have negative impacts by reducing the micronutrient availability.

7 VITAMINS

There are two classes of vitamins: fat-soluble and water-soluble. Both classes are organic, the major difference is in the name. They are either hydrophobic or hydrophilic. Hydrophobic vitamins are fat-soluble and hydrophilic vitamins are water-soluble. That means they are either compatible with fat-based or water-based substances. The fat-soluble vitamins are A, D, E, and K, and the water-soluble vitamins are B vitamins (B1, B2, B3, B5, B6, B9, and B12), vitamin C, biotin, and choline. Vitamins don't supply calories, but they all have specific functions. They are found in different foods and in different amounts. Just like the macronutrients, too much or too little will have an impact on the body, but in the case of vitamins and minerals it is being deficient or toxic instead of gaining or losing weight.

In general the water-soluble vitamins are known as co-enzymes, which means they are organic enzyme helpers. Their biggest roles are in assisting energy metabolism. The big three are B1 (thiamin), B2 (riboflavin), and B3 (niacin). They are highly associated with macronutrient metabolism and therefore essential to cellular energy production. That does not mean the others are of less importance. They are all essential to maintaining healthy conditions and an efficiently operating body of systems. For example, vitamin B12, which is found in meat, has essential functions such as helping cells make DNA, helping cells metabolize protein and fat, and promoting the health of nerve cells, red blood cells, and other cells in the body. So you can see all of the water-soluble vitamins are important, and getting the right amount is essential to health and function and may even have implications for performance.

Just like the water-solubles, the fat-soluble vitamins have specific functions, but they are not as directly involved in energy metabolism. Because they are hydrophobic they act a lot like a fat molecule. In fact, their backbone is very similar to a fat molecule's. Some even provide the building blocks for the body to make steroid hormones like testosterone and the estrogens. These vitamins have roles that range from blood clotting and anti-clotting to facilitating bone mineral deposition and promoting general cellular health via anti-oxidant action. These reasons are why getting the appropriate amounts is crucial.

Vitamins are present in a wide range of foods. Some foods hold higher concentrations, while others may not have any of that same nutrient. This is why it can be harmful to completely cut an entire food type from your intake. All naturally existing food types provide benefits to the human body in the form of some type of nutrient availability. Also, limiting your intake to one type of food can be harmful because there is no benefit to consuming excess nutrients while liming others, if you have ever heard overfed but undernourished then you are aware of this concept. The body can only use so much of one nutrient, and in excess you can reach a point of toxicity. This also applies to minerals, and because minerals are metals an excess that leads to toxicity can be more dangerous.

8 MINERALS

Minerals are nutrients that the body requires in even smaller amounts than vitamins. Just like vitamins, they do not supply any energy. There is a reason foods are enriched with calcium and other minerals, like iodine in table salt. They are inorganic substances that help enzymes, and therefore called co-factors. Since they are metals they are more dangerous in larger amounts, but it is more common to be deficient than in excess.

Different minerals are found in a variety of foods, in different concentrations just like other nutrients. Each has a specific function within the body, and are required in different amounts. Based on the required amounts there are two classifications, micro- and macro-minerals.

Minerals' roles include providing electrical charges to cellular membranes, acting as synergists in muscle contraction, water balance, delivering oxygen, immune function, metabolic regulation, and a whole host of other functions. This is why getting the appropriate amounts of this class of nutrient is crucial to good health. The same concept of not limiting food sources and not excluding food sources applies to mineral availability. You want to ensure you are getting everything you need out of your nutritional intake.

9 WATER

Most people learned in school that water is composed of two hydrogen atoms and one oxygen atom: H_2O. But what is the significance of that chemical make-up, and why does the human body require so much of it?

First, the adult body is composed of approximately 60% water, and we know that the body is constantly performing chemical reactions using water, so it must be replenished. Water regulates our body temperature as the chemical reactions occurring in the body create heat. Oxygen has an energy (electron) attracting quality and displays it in the final steps of aerobic energy production. This is important because during aerobic exercise that process is the main mechanism utilized to keep the muscles energized. On top of this, the body requires water in order to move substances efficiently, and for the systems in the body to work together to maintain life and provide a balanced environment.

There are two main fluid compartments in the body. The first is the Intracellular Fluid or ICF, which makes up the majority of the body's water at approximately 70%. The second is the Extracellular Fluid, or ECF, which makes up the remaining 30%.

The ICF and ECF are the water compartments of the body. The ICF is the fluid that is retained within each individual cell, of which there are trillions. The ECF is all of the fluid outside of the cells. That includes blood, cerebral spinal fluid, digestive juices, joint fluid, and all other water-based fluids.

In regards to exercise, the skeletal muscle is approximately 75% water. The joints that facilitate the movement made by those muscles also use a water-based fluid. This fluid is known as synovial fluid, and it provides lubrication for efficient movement of those joints. You can see that water, at a minimum, is important for life, and why it's important to stay hydrated when exercising. When we consider that the action of metabolizing macronutrients creates heat, i.e. burning calories, we can understand why the muscle is made of so much water, especially since it is the most metabolically active tissue.

During a one-day period men should be consuming about 16 cups of water and women about 13 [65]. This is based on men generally having more lean mass, specifically muscle, requiring more water for optimal function of that muscle tissue. Women naturally have a higher body fat percentage due to biological parameters, which means on the grand perspective a smaller percentage of their total mass is skeletal muscle.

Daily water intake comes from beverages and food. The more exercise performed, the greater the amount of water your body will require to ensure you don't offset water balance or cause dehydration. These numbers are recommendations for healthy conditions. Water is found in most foods and fluids, but keep in mind the more you replace other fluids with water the more unnecessary sugars and other ingredients you are removing from your intake. If your concern is health these can be important considerations to be made.

Hydration is about both water intake and electrolyte balance, so ensuring the water that is lost through sweat and increased breath rate is replaced is crucial, as is replacing the electrolytes that are lost during exercise. If exercise goes over one hour or is performed at a very high intensity, a sport drink that is composed of six to eight percent carbohydrate and contains electrolytes can be consumed to increase fuel availability and help replace lost electrolytes [66].

Electrolytes are molecules that provide positive and negative attraction, they are salts (minerals). For example, table salt is made up of Sodium and Chloride, NaCl. In water, these molecules are separated and regain the original charges that brought them together in the first place, sodium is positive and chloride is negative (Na^+ and Cl^-). Once inside the body these electrolytes facilitate bodily functions in their designated fluid compartments.

10 ALCOHOL

We know that there are three macronutrients, and those are nutrients which the human body metabolizes for the purpose of producing cellular energy. There is actually a fourth macronutrient, or pseudo-macronutrient, that provides energy when broken down.

When fats, carbohydrates, and proteins are metabolized they go through cellular processes that start in a place within the cell called the cytosol or cytoplasm. Cytosol is the cells' water-based, jelly-like filling that holds all of its components in place. The cell has its own version of organs, they are called organelles. One of those is the mitochondria, which is the energy harvester. The mitochondria takes the metabolites of macronutrients through a couple of processes and turns them into ATP (Adenosine Triphosphate), a molecule that the cell uses to power all action, and coined energy currency. There are two ways the cells metabolize nutrients -- in the cytosol and in the mitochondria, anaerobically and aerobically. Anaerobic means it does not require oxygen to perform, while aerobic does. These processes are what carbohydrates, fats, and proteins go through. However, there is another place and process used for the fourth macronutrient.

The title of this chapter identifies the fourth macronutrient, alcohol or ethanol. In regards to the body's biology, there are substances that cause damage which the body is not designed to handle, at least in high amounts. These are heavy metals, drugs, and poisons. They all can be considered biological toxins. This may sound odd considering the prevalence of alcohol in today's society, however, if we look at the body from the biological perspective, becoming intoxicated is actually a symptom of ethanol poisoning. Too much ethanol consumed too quickly will cause death via ethanol's impacts on the body's homeostatic conditions, namely the pH or acid-base balance. In the metabolism of ethanol, acetaldehyde is one of the major byproducts of liver's processing [67]. It is acidic and has a huge impact on the body's pH.

Recall one of the roles of the liver is to filter out toxins. The liver is structurally designed for filtration and processing. The cells in the liver are called hepatocytes. As alcohol, or any toxin or nutrient, reaches the liver through the blood, the hepatocytes begin this processing and filtration. In the presence of excessive alcohol intake, the processing and filtration cannot work fast enough. Therefore, the alcohol circulates in the blood until it can be processed correctly. That is why it takes time for alcohol's effect to wear off, and why a damaged liver is one of the major characteristics of chronic alcohol consumption. The hepatocytes become overworked from the constant demand.

Most consider beer, wine, liquor, or other choice of drink to contain the standard carbohydrate energy source. This may even be why many pay attention to carbs on the label. However, it is the alcohol that influences metabolism more than the carbohydrates. Once you ingest a drink your body immediately tags it as a priority. It does this to get the recognized toxin out of it as soon as it can.

The body does not want it so it begins to break it down. This cannot be done fast enough through the traditional processes, so an additional metabolic pathway is utilized to assist. This pathway is performed in an organelle called the Endoplasmic Reticulum (ER) of the cell. The significance of this is that it does not take place where the metabolism of other macronutrients does. Once it is complete the products do go into the normal pathways for harvesting ATP; in this we can see that the body is using whatever it can to break down the ethanol and get rid of it as fast as it can using whatever it can. This pathway is called MEOS, or Microsomal Ethanol Oxidizing System. The metabolites of this pathway are even more toxic to the body than the primary breakdown of ethanol [67], which includes but is not limited to acetaldehyde production, acidosis, high sugar, high insulin, and increased free-radical production.

Recall carbohydrates and proteins have four calories per gram, while fat has nine calories per gram. In recognizing alcohol goes through energy metabolism, we are also recognizing it has calories. In fact, alcohol contains more calories than carbohydrates and proteins. Alcohol contains seven calories per gram. That means that the pathways which process this pseudo-macronutrient are very significant, not just in health but also in energy balance. To put this into perspective, a twelve-ounce beer that is five percent alcohol contains roughly seventeen grams of alcohol. That means that beer has about 119 calories just from alcohol. An eight-ounce glass of wine that is eleven percent alcohol has roughly twenty-five grams of alcohol. That means it has about 175 calories just from alcohol. And a mixed drink that contains an eighty-proof spirit of one and a half ounces contains about seventeen grams of alcohol, which equates to roughly 119 calories just from alcohol. When considering your caloric intake you cannot discount alcohol. These calories can quickly add up, especially during a night of drinking.

Even when the diet fulfills what the body needs, alcohol consumption causes acute [68] and even chronic dysregulation of nutrient absorption. This dysregulation of nutrient processing is hugely impactful on anyone, and we must consider that the cell and the body are always in a state of reacting in response to their environment. This is what homeostasis is, the whole body creating conditions that allow survival of a stimulus or change.

When the body is forced to prioritize alcohol, even if there are other nutrients that need processing, there is really only one option, putting everything else on hold which can mean storage of energy. There is also impaired absorption and utilization of macro and micronutrients. The biggest impact is on the liver. With its key role in maintaining amino acids, glucose, fats, and many other blood constituents, the damaging effects of chronic and excessive alcohol consumption are huge on health status.

With the understanding of how alcohol consumption impacts metabolism, we can start to look at how alcohol impacts other factors of the body's health. When ordering a drink in a social environment or a restaurant, most people don't typically crave the healthy food. And even if they did, the majority of places that serve alcohol don't usually have an extensive set of healthier options. This is because they know that people will crave fried, unhealthy foods and they want to capitalize on those cravings.

Just as alcohol impacts metabolism, it also impacts other parts of the body's normal functioning. A good majority of hunger and satiety are controlled by hormones. When the hormone ghrelin is released we feel hungry, and when leptin is released it provides the feeling of satiation and fullness [69]. Alcohol interferes with the body's ability to regulate these by never stopping the release of ghrelin when you begin eating and not releasing leptin to make you feel full. The regulation of hunger is more complicated than this, but as you can see alcohol, at a minimum has a negative impact on hunger dynamics.

It also impacts cravings, and this is why when you are drinking you are more inclined to order a cheeseburger and fries or loaded nachos over a grilled chicken salad with the dressing on the side. It factors in to why you eat more than you typically would before becoming full. So not only does it have a big impact on total calorie intake. It could manifest in snacking where you eat an entire bag of chips, pretzels, or other snacks. A lot of this has to do with individual factors and the social environment as well.

On top of all of this, the body's ability to regulate blood sugar is dependent on specific hormones. The main hormones are insulin and glucagon. There are others involved in the dynamic process, but these two are the most significant. They help the body use sugar and keep the proper amount in the blood. Alcohol may acutely change the body's ability to do this by negatively influencing insulin sensitivity [70].

Another process that is highly controlled by hormones is water balance. The hangover goes hand-in-hand with any range of alcohol consumption. It is a result of dehydration and electrolyte imbalance. When alcohol goes through the body, among the many places it reaches are the kidneys. There it influences water and electrolyte balance [71], which causes dehydration. The body doesn't reabsorb water when it is supposed to, and this is why when drinking you are constantly finding your way to the restroom.

To add to all of those influences, alcohol also impacts the digestive system's ability to absorb nutrients. As food goes through the body it is broken down and the nutrients are absorbed in specific areas of the digestive tract. With alcohol introduced to the equation, nutrients are broken down and never absorbed, or absorption is impaired in some manner at the time of consumption [72]. This malabsorption has even been found to continue after the initial ingestion of alcohol in a chronic manner [73].

One of the major impacts this malabsorption leads to is a decrease in calcium and other minerals in the body. When minerals like calcium are not absorbed from the diet, the body has to resort to its stored deposits, the bones, which can cause a reduced bone mineral density. This is most significant in long-term, excessive consumption; however alcohol does cause malabsorption anytime it is ingested.

Reduced bone mineral density is a process that occurs naturally with age, but can be made worse by chronic alcohol consumption. Calcium is not the only nutrient that is affected. Alcohol consumption negatively impacts all gut absorption dynamics, which significantly impacts the body's tissues, and in chronic excess has been found to affect the functionality of the liver and brain [72]. In regards to the brain, alcohol has its most significant impact on neurodegeneration and causing brain cell death [74].

Hormones that impact the metabolism, hunger, satiety, cravings, water balance, and blood sugar are not the only ones that alcohol consumption negatively impacts. Sex hormones, or androgens, are also impacted. Alcohol can impact estrogen and testosterone levels in both males and females. In males, excessive alcohol consumption causes the liver to metabolize the circulating testosterone and bring levels down [75]. It has also been found to decrease testicular size and gonadal function in overconsumption [76]. This decreases fertility and sexual performance, and has implications for other issues brought on by low testosterone levels. In women, acute alcohol consumption has been found to increase the circulating estradiol [78], the primary estrogen. Chronic consumption may increase the likelihood for the development of breast cancer [78]. In general, the sex hormones are negatively impacted, in both males and females. There are many other factors that must be considered, but changing hormone levels via alcohol consumption (especially chronic and excessive) has been shown to promote negative impacts on the biological systems of the body.

One final consideration for alcohol's impact on the body is in association to protein synthesis and the process of protein turnover. Protein turnover was brought up earlier, but to go into a little more detail, it is the opposing processes of Muscle Protein Synthesis (MPS) and Muscle Protein Breakdown (MPB). The body is constantly in a state of protein turnover, making new proteins to replace old ones. This is especially important in the context of exercise. To be in a positive state of protein balance you have to be performing greater MPS than MPB. With alcohol in the equation, MPS is essentially not happening. There is a stream of processes in the cell that occur to result in new muscle protein, and alcohol interferes with them. They go to a certain point, then alcohol jumps in and keeps the final steps from occurring [79]. This is hugely impactful when the body is adapting to exercise by enhancing MPS. Essentially it means new muscle isn't built when alcohol is consumed.

Now that you understand what that beer, glass of wine, or mixed drink does to your cellular metabolism and body, what does that mean for your overall goal attainment?

The most important thing to consider is that the phrase "everything in moderation" applies here. Are there bad things about alcohol consumption? Yes, but in moderation there could be benefits. Some studies suggest that one glass of red wine per day may provide decreased risk for all-cause mortality, cardiovascular events, stroke, peripheral arterial disease, and congestive heart failure, as well as improved gut health [80, 81].

Even if some benefits have been found, if fat loss is your goal then alcohol may be your enemy. Also, chronic and excessive alcohol consumption provides negative outcomes to all. As with most foods and drinks, remember "everything in moderation."

11 SUGARS AND CHEAT DAYS

Earlier we discussed how combinations of sugars derived from carbohydrates can be important in the context of energy and health. Refined sugars are short sugar molecules that are added to foods to increase the sweetness and appeal to the consumer. Even though sugars are all the same composition of elements, it is the glycemic impact of the short, refined sugars on the body and the lack of other nutrients that makes them different.

The first thing to remember is the Glycemic Index (GI). A more refined or shorter sugar generally does not cause the same insulin reaction as a low GI food. They are both absorbed at about the same rate, but the high GI food does not signal insulin to help clear that new sugar out of the blood to the extent the low GI food does. This can be damaging to the body in certain contexts.

One of the problems with added and refined sugars is that they dramatically influence the blood's sugar level. It is also important to understand that the body cells can only store and take up so much sugar, so if they are full they will not take in any more. This leaves the blood levels high and increases the risk for damage. Because the cells are already at capacity, they can reject the insulin and leave the sugar in the blood, but the body still wants to bring that blood sugar down. That means the pancreas may continue to pump out insulin in an attempt to lower blood sugar, which stresses the cells that make it. This causes high sugar and insulin blood levels. If this is continued over time it can be extremely detrimental and is part of how insulin resistance is developed. It can also play into the development of Type-II diabetes [82]. But, this is really only the case when there is limited exercise to assist in using the sugar.

When the cells require more insulin to take in the same amount of sugar, they have begun the development of insulin resistance. The development of insulin resistance is why a high-sugar diet is a major contributor to developing Type-II diabetes. If insulin resistance is continued, the cells that make the insulin will start to exhaust themselves and won't be able to produce the amount of insulin needed to regulate blood sugar. When that happens the body is no longer able to control its blood sugar, and blood tests will show impaired blood sugar regulation.

The development of Type-II diabetes can be highly dependent on diet (*and exercise*), as ingested carbohydrates are directly tied to insulin output by the pancreas. The development of the condition is very complicated, with a lot of factors at play. In fact, Type-II diabetes can take over ten years to develop [82]. That said, blood sugar levels are not the most accurate way of testing for it. As insulin resistance is how the body starts its path to this type of diabetes, the blood insulin levels can be the best way to test. If your cells require more insulin to handle the same amount of sugar, it can mean that your body is secreting extra insulin to compensate for the insulin resistance, and therefore insulin dynamics are out of whack.

Sugar molecules are sharp and sticky, and the vessels that transport blood to the tissues containing these molecules can be very small and have many branching points. This provides an endless amount of places for these sugar molecules to cause damage. Any damage causes the body to begin repair. When those damaged areas are repaired, a certain cascade of events allows that area to be susceptible to plaque and cholesterol buildup, and set the stage for the development of atherosclerosis [83]. This cascade that starts with that initial damage is followed by the body's inflammatory response to fix the issue, and ends with LDL cholesterol accumulation in the area. This explanation makes it sound simple, however it is a complicated process where the body is trying to fortify the damaged area to prevent further damage. Ultimately this can narrow the vessel, which increases local blood pressure and risk for many other complicated vascular conditions.

A diet that includes high added or refined sugars may not seem like such a bad thing, but you must remember that all the little things you put into your body impact you on a cellular level. What you see in the mirror does not always reflect your health. Remember, if it impacts you on a cellular level, and you have trillions of cells, then the impact is not on a small scale.

Many times people criticize the consumption of fruit because of the high amounts of sugar. What is coming into play here is the Glycemic Index. Some fruits are considered high on the index, but they are very nutrient dense. Consider one serving of banana versus one serving of gummy bears. They are both high on the index, but one is nutrient dense while the other is not. You must remember the sugar in fruit comes with many other nutrients. Eating fruit (no matter the GI rating) adds vitamins, minerals, phytochemicals, fiber, anti-oxidants, and other needed nutrients to your intake. For reasons like this, the index cannot be used to asses a carbohydrate's impact on your health. It should, however, be used to understand the amplitude of the insulin reaction that the carbohydrate food has [36, 37, 38, 84]. If you are not saturating your body with unnecessary added sugars and using the energy you put in your body, the amount of sugar in fruits will not impact you negatively.

There are many ways to label a sugar. For example, any syrup, fruit concentrate, fruit juice, molasses, or natural sugar are also added sugars that are sometimes disguised in food labeling. Do not forget that most naturally occurring sugars end with -ose. Of particular significance is fructose, including high fructose corn syrup (HFCS), a common form of fructose associated with negative impacts. There was once an idea that HFCS was independent in its negative impact on body composition and hunger, but research supports that any fructose has the same negative impact, including table sugar (regular sucrose) [85 – 88]. This is because HFCS only contains 5% greater fructose than table sugar. Normal table sugar is 50% fructose and 50% glucose, while HFCS is 55% fructose and 45% glucose.

The impact referenced is that this type of sugar does not stimulate the leptin-ghrelin response where ghrelin is suppressed and leptin is released. In normal ingestion those things do happen, and hunger is suppressed and the feeling of satiation or fullness is felt. At any rate, sugar can be dangerous, especially ingested as liquid calories, and should be limited due to the potential to add to the development of obesity, Type-II diabetes, and metabolic disease [89].

It is only normal to crave the high-sugar, high-salt, high-fat foods, and even your favorite drink. They taste good, are very accessible in our world today, and can provide stress relief. They can serve as a reward. They may also provide a large amount of calories that you could have already burned or accounted for in your plan. They can shock your body's systems because they are not used to them; specifically the gastrointestinal tract which includes the stomach, intestines, and the gut microbiome that live there. The microbiome is becoming recognized for its impact in biological whole-body health, function, and nutritional dynamics [90]. Because of that we need to understand that dramatic changes in dietary intake, the cheat meal, has a huge impact.

Everyone who has dieted has heard of the term cheat meal. They often have a negative connotation as a way to eat unhealthy. Instead, I like to look at it as a way of rewarding yourself for maintaining a healthy lifestyle and doing what needs to be done. Cheat meals may provide that metaphorical light at the end of the tunnel. There are many factors in society that make eating healthy and exercising regularly difficult. A reward to yourself is sometimes the best way to keep on track, and an alcoholic beverage or favorite treat can be a part of that reward.

One of the most significant things to consider when it comes to the cheat meal is that research indicates food addictions are comparative to addictive behaviors like drug abuse [91, 92]. There are differences in the mechanisms, but there are also similarities between the food and drug variations of addiction. Every time that high-sugar, salty, or fried food is chosen, the continuation of the behavior is allowed. The problem with having a cheat meal is that it keeps the foods that are addictive in the diet, which allows the continuation of those cravings. This is something that has to be accounted for.

Earlier we discussed the difficulties of creating an energy deficit, especially when you add a large amount of calories. Because of this, when you choose to have a cheat meal you are countering your fat loss and may add weight back that you may have lost. Even if you are exercising five days a week, you may not be doing enough to burn the calories you are adding back in on your cheat day or meal. That depends on how extreme of a cheat you have, but it is very possible to eat an enormous amount of calories on a cheat.

The cheat meal is another behavior to control. Maintaining the behavior of granting a cheat meal keeps the behavior of poor eating in your life. Keeping a bad behavior in your life has a great potential of causing issues in the future, like using this behavior as a fall back during a time of crisis or high stress. Considering the rebound, sugar addiction, and high calorie content in the typical cheat meal it may be especially bad for those people that are just starting off. It keeps the calories high, maintains addiction to the foods, and encourages the bad behavior of poor eating in their life.

Diets alone don't work unless they are part of an overall lifestyle. Doing something that is maintainable is the best way to make healthy eating behaviors last for the long-run. Giving yourself a reward helps, and for some that includes an alcoholic beverage or whatever you choose on occasion. However, the level of "cheating" has to be a part of the lifestyle that is in alignment with the long-term goal. Cheating gives you a way to eat healthy and not feel overwhelmed by an eating program that is full of things that at times you may not enjoy. Some people are able to go without, but it is up to you to find the right balance in your nutritional intake so that you can maintain your healthy lifestyle. Eating healthy in general is the goal. It is okay to stray occasionally, but it has to be in a way that won't cause you to binge.

All of this said, the idea behind the cheat is a good one -- keeping someone motivated. Although I challenge the cheat with flexibility. If you have a flexible plan that meets your needs you won't need to cheat. Food intake does have a relationship with endorphin release [93]. We must know that extremely limiting our food in some novel way that is pushed by an influencer is not the best; the best way for you is the way that you can maintain for the long term and gives your body what it needs.

12 DIETS AND KNOWING THE LABEL

The word diet, or the phrase, "I'm on a diet," is misused far too often. The word diet refers dietary intake. The term "going on a diet" is a misuse, because technically we are all on a "diet". The correct way to word it would be to say you're changing your dietary intake, words have more power than we realize. Many people think that the only way to obtain the weight they want is through a diet, and this has given "diet" a negative connotation. But, in reality this misuse will continue. Knowing this and that the word is referring to nutritional intake and not the commonly thought starvation or elimination of certain nutrients, we need to look at other aspects of nutrition. Understand that a healthy nutritional intake, dietary intake, or diet, needs to be balanced in order to fulfill your energy and nutrient requirements.

The word diet has created some marketability of certain food products to fit what people want to consume while "on a diet." We have all heard or seen marketing and advertising for sugar-free, fat-free, and organic food industry marketing. In this chapter we'll look into why these three are such a focus.

Sugar-Free

There are many negative impacts that can come with a high-sugar diet due to its association with the development of metabolic dysregulation. Earlier we discussed some of the dynamics of the development of Type-II diabetes and how sugar plays a role in that. Sugar glycosylates cells and other biological components. Glycosylation is simply the word used to describe sugar coating. This occurs in normal functioning, but in high levels it is extremely damaging. In this example high blood sugar seems to have a specific impact on male reproductive dynamics, impairing ability and lowering testosterone levels [94]. This is just one more example of the negative impacts that a diet high in sugar can have, but don't forget that food and its energy is there to fuel the body so exercise needs to be factored into this equation. These many examples have opened the door to marketability of the reduction of sugar in food-like products and the food production industry.

Marketers take advantage of our knowledge that high-sugar diets can be harmful, but we must ask questions about this marketing attempt on our food intake. If a food product is labeled "sugar-free" and truly does not contain sugar, how is it sweet? These products may contain artificial sweeteners, and the most common of those seem to be sugar alcohols. These end in the suffix -itol instead of –ose, like sugars. Examples include lacitol, xylitol, and maltitol. They are derived from fruits and vegetables, but are not completely a sugar and not completely an alcohol. Their chemical make-up resembles both, but there are differences. As they are not a sugar they do not have the same effect on blood glucose and therefore do not elicit the same insulin reaction [95]. They provide the sweet taste without causing the same negative impacts that traditional sugars do.

Since they are not metabolized the same way as a sugar they affect the body differently. Specifically, they are not totally absorbed and they tend to be sweeter than traditional sugars. Once they pass through the upper portion of the digestive system, where other nutrients are absorbed, they continue to the large intestines and are passed out of the body with the rest of the waste. While they are in this part of the digestive system they actually ferment due to their chemical structure. This produces gas and has the possibility of causing digestive complications, especially in people that have sensitive digestive systems. The more consumed, the more likely these complications are to occur.

Sugar alcohols are somewhat new, and their long-term effects are not totally understood. This is just one of the reasons why it is important to understand there are inherent risks when putting something in your body, and specifically for sugar alcohols why you should be careful of excessive amounts and the timing of ingestion. The following are some examples: xylitol, malitol, erythritol, sorbitol, mannitol, isomalt, lactitol, and polyglycitol.

Fat-Free

"Fat-free" marketing and food production is based on the goal of reducing fat intake in the general public. It has been communicated that fat was the cause of many health issues, which led to this specific type of food production in order to target individuals who wanted to enjoy their favorite foods with less fat content.

A fat-free food may seem like a good choice, but how is it that a food that once had fat in it now has none? Another question to ask is knowing that fat does have important biological roles, why should we be looking to foods that are processed even further to remove the nutrient? Processed being the key word.

Fat-free, food-like product labeling is an effective marketing tool. But ask yourself, are those foods really healthy? We have already looked at the effect of sugar on the body and how too much can create health risks for the consumer. Even so, sugar makes food taste sweet and adds flavor. It also stimulates the release of hormones, which make us feel euphoric and happy after eating them. The same is true with fats. This is the case because we are programmed to seek foods that are calorie dense in case of a time when food is scarce, and because of that eating foods with fats makes us feel happy and we tend to crave them. If you were to remove the fat from a food, how would it taste? Probably not very good, which means a product like that would not sell very well. Therefore, food manufacturers found ways to make fat-free products taste good even while not containing fat or containing less fat.

Sugar is one way, but not the only way, to replace unsaturated, saturated, and trans-fats. There are fat substitutes that are built off of the different macronutrient molecules. They can be made out of proteins, carbohydrates, and even fat-based fat substitutes are used. They are designed so that the term fat-free could be used to market the product, as technically the food product does not contain a traditional dietary fat.

Fat substitutes provide the same satisfaction that fat provides in the form of that creamy, full taste. But, depending on what the substitute is made of, it can still have a significant amount of calories. If it is built from a carbohydrate source it can have anywhere from zero to four calories per gram. Protein-based fat substitutes have four calories per gram. The fat substitutes that are made of fat can contain anywhere from zero to nine calories per gram. The variation in calorie harvest depends on the processing and fat-substitute base.

A food product that says it does not contain fat might still have some form of fat that is described differently on the label. And just because it claims to be fat-free doesn't mean it contains less calories. This is why it is important is to read everything on the label and know that fat-free labeling may not be telling you what you think it is. On the positive side, some things that have a fat-free label never contained fat. This is another reason why reading the label is so important. There could be a similar product made by a different company that costs less because they don't push the fat-free labeling.

Fat-based fat substitutes can be listed as Duro-Lo, Salatrim, or Olean. They are often used in baked goods, confection goods, and savory snacks. They provide the fatty-like mouth feel and water retention like typical dietary fat. Duro-Lo has 9 caloreis per gram, Salatrim has 5 calories per gram, and Olean doesn't have any calories [96].

Carbohydrate-based fat substitutes can be listed as Beta-Trim, Avicel Cellulose Gel, Slendid, Litesse, and STA-SLIM. They are often used in baked goods, processed meats, spreads, sauces, dairy products, frozen deserts, salad dressings, cookies, gum, frostings, and fillings. They provide the fatty-like mouth feel, water retention, are used for gelling and thickener, and add bulk to the food-like product. Beta-Trim and STA-SLIM can have 1-4 calories per gram, Litesse has 1 calorie per gam, and Avicel Cellulose Gel and Slendid don't have any calories [96].

There is one protein-based fat substitute, listed as Simplesse. It is often used in dairy products, salad dressings, and spreads. It provides the full mouth feel and can have anywhere from 1-4 calories per gram [96].

Organic

Organic Labeling is regulated by the USDA like all other food labeling. The USDA has set specific guidelines that companies have to abide by in order to have the organic label. But many people also equate organic foods with healthier diets. Are the organic foods really as good for you as you think?

First we must know what allows the company to label a food or food product with each specific label type. The label types include no designation of organic materials, Made with Organic Ingredients, Organic, and 100% Organic.

The USDA uses standards to determine if an ingredient can be labeled organic. The standards are very intensive and in order for a food to carry the organic label, or any of the allowed derivatives, its preparation must follow the requirements set in the Code of Federal Regulations. These and other reasons are why organic foods are more expensive, however there is no evidence that shows organic foods are more nutritious than non-organic foods. Even so, it does not mean they aren't. The question is, should you spend your money on foods labeled organic, when you can get foods that contain the same nutrients for less money, but maybe with a few pesticides and fertilizers that you will wash off anyway?

Is there a need to buy into the marketing of those big companies trying to apply to your desire to eat healthier? If you really want to eat healthy and improve your impact on the environment, find a local farm that grows the things you need and has no need to have different labels for "Organic" and "Non-organic." Not only would you be improving your intake, but you are improving the quality of your local environment and economy.

USDA Organic Labeling		
Term Allowed	**Ingredient Parameters**	**Labeling Permitted**
100% Organic	All ingredients of the finished product are certified 100% organic	USDA Organic with seal
Organic	95% of finished product ingredients meet organic criteria	USDA Organic with seal
Made with Organic Ingredients	70% of finished product ingredients meet organic criteria	Made with Organic Ingredients
Contains Organic Ingredients	Less than 70% of finished product ingredients meet criteria	May only list Organic Ingredients on the information panel

ADAPTED FROM: CODE OF FEDERAL REGUALTIONS, TITLE 7, SUBTITILE B, CHAPTER I, SUBCHAPTER M, PART 205, SUBPART D, §205.301 PRODUCT COMPOSITION.

Understanding Food Labeling

Food labeling includes three basic ways for companies to market what the food item can do for the consumer. These include the nutrient content claims, health claims, and structure or function claims. These three types of labeling are found on almost every food item.

The nutrient content claims are labels such as fat-free, sugar-free, low-fat, low-sodium, high-fiber, or anything that describes what the food item has or does not have in it. It is simply a way to show an appealing nutrient content without the consumer having to read the nutrition label.

The next type of label is the health claim. This type of label has two parts. It lists the nutrient that is being called attention to and what potential benefit it has related to health for the consumer if they eat it. This would be when products have labels that say things like, "can help reduce risk of diabetes," "can lower cholesterol," "lowers risk of heart disease," "can help reduce blood pressure," or any similar statement.

The last food label type is the structure or function claim. The structure or function claim is the simplest labeling type. It only lists what a nutrient does in the human body. The nutrient usually exists in the competitors' product, but this label type calls attention to its natural function to catch the consumers' eye. This is when a food label tells the consumer that calcium builds strong bones, fiber promotes regular bowel movements, protein helps build muscle, B vitamins promote energy, unsaturated fats are heart healthy, or any other claim that gives the basic function of a nutrient. Because this type of labeling is the most basic, the structure and function claim do not have to be preapproved by the FDA like the other two, although they do have to be truthful.

The health claim requires research and proof, while the structure and function do not. This is because the health claims are actually telling the consumer of a benefit in promoting health, but the structure and function is defining what that nutrient does. Food labeling of this type is very effective and provides the consumer with truthful information. It is important to know that just because two similar products don't have the same label marketing they could still provide those same benefits or functions. It is important to read the nutritional information and understand what you are buying. You could purchase a different product that does the exact same thing and save yourself some money when healthfully shopping, instead of following the bright labels that want you to purchase the most expensive product.

One of the most notorious ways the sugar-free and fat-free diets are marketed is by using the content labeling method. If a food never contained sugar or fat, the label can read it is free of that ingredient. That is why at times you see a food product that has a label that reads "gluten free" even when the food never actually had gluten in it. However, that label caught your eye and you bought that product instead of the competitor's without the label. In fact, the product you bought could have cost more because they are boasting the gluten-free marketability. Make sure you know what you are looking for on a label. If it doesn't contain wheat or its derivatives, barley, or rye then chances are it doesn't contain gluten or it never did. Labeling a product is marketing of a product, so know what you are buying and putting on you and your family's plates.

| Nutrient | Labeling Terms | | | |
	Free	Low	Reduced or Less	Light
Calories (cal)	< 5 cal per serving	≤ 40 cal per serving	At least 25% fewer cal per serving	If the food contains 50% or more of its cal from fat, then the fat must be reduced by atleast 50%
Total Fat	< 0.5g per serving	≤ 3g per serving	At least 25% less fat per serving	If the food contains 50% or more of its cal from fat, then the fat must be reduced by atleast 50%
Saturated Fat	< 0.5g per serving	≤ 1g per serving	At least 25% less saturated fat per serving	N/A
Cholesterol	< 2mg per serving	≤ 20 mg per serving	At least 25% less cholesterol per serving	N/A
Sodium	<5mg per serving	< 140mg per serving	At least 25% less sodium per serving	If food is "Low Calorie" and "Low Fat" and sodium is reduced by at least 50%.
Sugars	<0.5g	N/A	At least 25% less sugar per serving	N/A

ADAPTED FROM: FOOD AND DRUG ADMINISTRATION (2013). A FOOD LABELING GUIDE: GUIDANCE FOR INDUSTRY. U.S. DEPARTMENT OF HEALTH AND HUMAN SERVICES. P. 87-90.

REFERENCES

1) ZOBEL, E. H., ET AL. (2016). "GLOBAL CHANGES IN FOOD SUPPLY AND THE OBESITY EPIDEMIC." CURR OBES REP 5(4): 449-455.

2) ZHAO, Y., ET AL. (2017). "FAST FOOD CONSUMPTION AND ITS ASSOCIATIONS WITH OBESITY AND HYPERTENSION AMONG CHILDREN: RESULTS FROM THE BASELINE DATA OF THE CHILDHOOD OBESITY STUDY IN CHINA MEGA-CITIES." BMC PUBLIC HEALTH 17(1): 933

3) ZHANG, N., ET AL. (2017). "CURRENT LIFESTYLE FACTORS THAT INCREASE RISK OF T2DM IN CHINA." EUR J CLIN NUTR 71(7): 832-838.

4) PADILLA, P. AND P. MIRAMONTES (2006). "A THEORETICAL FRAMEWORK FOR DEFINING SOME CONCEPTS IN EVOLUTION." RIV BIOL 99(2): 273-285.

5) BLAIR, S. N., ET AL. (1989). "PHYSICAL FITNESS AND ALL-CAUSE MORTALITY. A PROSPECTIVE STUDY OF HEALTHY MEN AND WOMEN." JAMA 262(17): 2395-2401.

6) BEAUMAN, C., ET AL. (2005). "THE PRINCIPLES, DEFINITION AND DIMENSIONS OF THE NEW NUTRITION SCIENCE." PUBLIC HEALTH NUTR 8(6A): 695-698.

7) PERRY, A. C., ET AL. (1997). "FITNESS, DIET AND CORONARY RISK FACTORS IN A SAMPLE OF SOUTHEASTERN U.S. CHILDREN." APPL HUMAN SCI 16(4): 133-141.

8) OTTEN, J. J., ET AL. (2006). DIETARY REFERENCE INTAKES: THE ESSENTIAL GUIDE TO NUTRIENT REQUIREMENTS, NATIONAL ACADEMIES PRESS.

9) BROOKS, G. A. AND J. MERCIER (1994). "BALANCE OF CARBOHYDRATE AND LIPID UTILIZATION DURING EXERCISE: THE "CROSSOVER" CONCEPT." J APPL PHYSIOL (1985) 76(6): 2253-2261.

10) CAREY, D. G. (2009). "QUANTIFYING DIFFERENCES IN THE "FAT BURNING" ZONE AND THE AEROBIC ZONE: IMPLICATIONS FOR TRAINING." J STRENGTH COND RES 23(7): 2090-2095.

11) NORTON, L. E., ET AL. (2009). "THE LEUCINE CONTENT OF A COMPLETE MEAL DIRECTS PEAK ACTIVATION BUT NOT DURATION OF SKELETAL MUSCLE PROTEIN SYNTHESIS AND MAMMALIAN TARGET OF RAPAMYCIN SIGNALING IN RATS." J NUTR 139(6): 1103-1109.

12) ANTHONY, J. C., ET AL. (2000). "LEUCINE STIMULATES TRANSLATION INITIATION IN SKELETAL MUSCLE OF POSTABSORPTIVE RATS VIA A RAPAMYCIN-SENSITIVE PATHWAY." J NUTR 130(10): 2413-2419.

13) NORTON, L. E. AND D. K. LAYMAN (2006). "LEUCINE REGULATES TRANSLATION INITIATION OF PROTEIN SYNTHESIS IN SKELETAL MUSCLE AFTER EXERCISE." J NUTR 136(2): 533S-537S

14) WATERLOW, J. C., ET AL. (1978). "PROTEIN TURNOVER IN MAN MEASURED WITH 15N: COMPARISON OF END PRODUCTS AND DOSE REGIMES." AM J PHYSIOL 235(2): E165-174.

15) BIOLO, G. (2013). "PROTEIN METABOLISM AND REQUIREMENTS." WORLD REV NUTR DIET 105: 12-20.

16) POTIER, M., ET AL. (2009). "PROTEIN, AMINO ACIDS AND THE CONTROL OF FOOD INTAKE." CURR OPIN CLIN NUTR METAB CARE 12(1): 54-58.

17) SANDERS, K., ET AL. (1994). "THE EFFECT OF DIETARY FAT LEVEL AND QUALITY ON PLASMA LIPOPROTEIN LIPIDS AND PLASMA FATTY ACIDS IN NORMOCHOLESTEROLEMIC SUBJECTS." LIPIDS 29(2): 129-138.

18) HENNING, A. L., ET AL. (2016). "CONSUMPTION OF A HIGH-FAT MEAL WAS ASSOCIATED WITH AN INCREASE IN MONOCYTE ADHESION MOLECULES, SCAVENGER RECEPTORS, AND PROPENSITY TO FORM FOAM CELLS." CYTOMETRY B CLIN CYTOM.

19) LIU, A. G., ET AL. (2017). "A HEALTHY APPROACH TO DIETARY FATS: UNDERSTANDING THE SCIENCE AND TAKING ACTION TO REDUCE CONSUMER CONFUSION." NUTR J 16(1): 53.

20) NATIONAL RESEARCH COUNCIL (NRC). RECOMMENDED DIETARY ALLOWANCES, 10TH ED. WASHINGTON, DC: NATIONAL ACADEMY OF SCIENCES; 1989.

21) POEHLMAN, E. T. (1989). "A REVIEW: EXERCISE AND ITS INFLUENCE ON RESTING ENERGY METABOLISM IN MAN." MED SCI SPORTS EXERC 21(5): 515-525.

22) HASSON, R. E., ET AL. (2011). "ACCURACY OF FOUR RESTING METABOLIC RATE PREDICTION EQUATIONS: EFFECTS OF SEX, BODY MASS INDEX, AGE, AND RACE/ETHNICITY." J SCI MED SPORT 14(4): 344-351.

23) TAI, M. M., ET AL. (1991). "MEAL SIZE AND FREQUENCY: EFFECT ON THE THERMIC EFFECT OF FOOD." AM J CLIN NUTR 54(5): 783-787.

24) ROY, B. D., ET AL. (1997). "EFFECT OF GLUCOSE SUPPLEMENT TIMING ON PROTEIN METABOLISM AFTER RESISTANCE TRAINING." J APPL PHYSIOL (1985) 82(6): 1882-1888.

25) CLEVELAND, B. M. AND G. M. WEBER (2010). "EFFECTS OF INSULIN-LIKE GROWTH FACTOR-I, INSULIN, AND LEUCINE ON PROTEIN TURNOVER AND UBIQUITIN LIGASE EXPRESSION IN RAINBOW TROUT PRIMARY MYOCYTES." AM J PHYSIOL REGUL INTEGR COMP PHYSIOL 298(2): R341-350.

26) DE CASTRO, J. M. (1993). "GENETIC INFLUENCES ON DAILY INTAKE AND MEAL PATTERNS OF HUMANS." PHYSIOL BEHAV 53(4): 777-782.

27) REDD, M. AND J. M. DE CASTRO (1992). "SOCIAL FACILITATION OF EATING: EFFECTS OF SOCIAL INSTRUCTION ON FOOD INTAKE." PHYSIOL BEHAV 52(4): 749-754.

28) ELLISTON, K. G., ET AL. (2017). "PERSONAL AND SITUATIONAL PREDICTORS OF EVERYDAY SNACKING: AN APPLICATION OF TEMPORAL SELF-REGULATION THEORY." BR J HEALTH PSYCHOL 22(4): 854-871.

29) PETROWSKI, K., ET AL. (2014). "CHEWING AFTER STRESS: PSYCHOSOCIAL STRESS INFLUENCES CHEWING FREQUENCY, CHEWING EFFICACY, AND APPETITE." PSYCHONEUROENDOCRINOLOGY 48: 64-76.

30) MASTROCOLA, R., ET AL. (2016). "HIGH-FRUCTOSE INTAKE AS RISK FACTOR FOR NEURODEGENERATION: KEY ROLE FOR CARBOXY METHYLLYSINE ACCUMULATION IN MICE HIPPOCAMPAL NEURONS." NEUROBIOL DIS 89: 65-75.

31) DE STEFANIS, D., ET AL. (2017). "EFFECTS OF CHRONIC SUGAR CONSUMPTION ON LIPID ACCUMULATION AND AUTOPHAGY IN THE SKELETAL MUSCLE." EUR J NUTR 56(1): 363-373.

32) GLIEMANN, L., ET AL. (2017). "ENDOTHELIAL MECHANOTRANSDUCTION PROTEINS AND VASCULAR FUNCTION ARE ALTERED BY DIETARY SUCROSE SUPPLEMENTATION IN HEALTHY YOUNG MALE SUBJECTS." J PHYSIOL 595(16): 5557-5571.

33) MACDONALD, I. A. (1999). "CARBOHYDRATE AS A NUTRIENT IN ADULTS: RANGE OF ACCEPTABLE INTAKES." EUR J CLIN NUTR 53 SUPPL 1: S101-106.

34) POTTER, M., ET AL. (2016). "THE WARBURG EFFECT: 80 YEARS ON." BIOCHEM SOC TRANS 44(5): 1499-1505.

35) ALEKSANDROVA, K., ET AL. (2017). "DIET, GUT MICROBIOME AND EPIGENETICS: EMERGING LINKS WITH INFLAMMATORY BOWEL DISEASES AND PROSPECTS FOR MANAGEMENT AND PREVENTION." NUTRIENTS 9(9).

36) EELDERINK, C., ET AL. (2012). "SLOWLY AND RAPIDLY DIGESTIBLE STARCHY FOODS CAN ELICIT A SIMILAR GLYCEMIC RESPONSE BECAUSE OF DIFFERENTIAL TISSUE GLUCOSE UPTAKE IN HEALTHY MEN." AM J CLIN NUTR 96(5): 1017-1024.

37) EELDERINK, C., ET AL. (2012). "THE GLYCEMIC RESPONSE DOES NOT REFLECT THE IN VIVO STARCH DIGESTIBILITY OF FIBER-RICH WHEAT PRODUCTS IN HEALTHY MEN." J NUTR 142(2): 258-263.

38) SCHAFER, G., ET AL. (2003). "COMPARISON OF THE EFFECTS OF DRIED PEAS WITH THOSE OF POTATOES IN MIXED MEALS ON POSTPRANDIAL GLUCOSE AND INSULIN CONCENTRATIONS IN PATIENTS WITH TYPE 2 DIABETES." AM J CLIN NUTR 78(1): 99-103.

39) SCHENK, S., ET AL. (2003). "DIFFERENT GLYCEMIC INDEXES OF BREAKFAST CEREALS ARE NOT DUE TO GLUCOSE ENTRY INTO BLOOD BUT TO GLUCOSE REMOVAL BY TISSUE." AM J CLIN NUTR 78(4): 742-748.

40) KAY, R. M. (1982). "DIETARY FIBER." J LIPID RES 23(2): 221-242.

41) FORIS, L. A. AND S. S. BHIMJI (2018). DIVERTICULOSIS. STATPEARLS. TREASURE ISLAND (FL).

42-43) CROWE, F. L., ET AL. (2011). "DIET AND RISK OF DIVERTICULAR DISEASE IN OXFORD COHORT OF EUROPEAN PROSPECTIVE INVESTIGATION INTO CANCER AND NUTRITION (EPIC): PROSPECTIVE STUDY OF BRITISH VEGETARIANS AND NON-VEGETARIANS." BMJ 343: D4131.

43) FLOCH, M. H. AND I. BINA (2004). "THE NATURAL HISTORY OF DIVERTICULITIS: FACT AND THEORY." J CLIN GASTROENTEROL 38(5 SUPPL 1): S2-7.

44) JASKIEWICZ, K., ET AL. (1986). "THE INFLUENCE OF DIET AND DIMETHYLHYDRAZINE ON THE SMALL AND LARGE INTESTINE OF VERVET MONKEYS." BR J EXP PATHOL 67(3): 361-369.

45) HIGGINS, J. A. (2004). "RESISTANT STARCH: METABOLIC EFFECTS AND POTENTIAL HEALTH BENEFITS." J AOAC INT 87(3): 761-768.

46) NGUYEN-DUY, T. B., ET AL. (2003). "VISCERAL FAT AND LIVER FAT ARE INDEPENDENT PREDICTORS OF METABOLIC RISK FACTORS IN MEN." AM J PHYSIOL ENDOCRINOL METAB 284(6): E1065-1071.

47) GASTALDELLI, A., ET AL. (2007). "RELATIONSHIP BETWEEN HEPATIC/VISCERAL FAT AND HEPATIC INSULIN RESISTANCE IN NONDIABETIC AND TYPE 2 DIABETIC SUBJECTS." GASTROENTEROLOGY 133(2): 496-506.

48) GERST, F., ET AL. (2017). "METABOLIC CROSSTALK BETWEEN FATTY PANCREAS AND FATTY LIVER: EFFECTS ON LOCAL INFLAMMATION AND INSULIN SECRETION." DIABETOLOGIA 60(11): 2240-2251.

49) ZINN, C., ET AL. (2017). "KETOGENIC DIET BENEFITS BODY COMPOSITION AND WELL-BEING BUT NOT PERFORMANCE IN A PILOT CASE STUDY OF NEW ZEALAND ENDURANCE ATHLETES." J INT SOC SPORTS NUTR 14: 22.

50) BURKE, L. M. (2015). "RE-EXAMINING HIGH-FAT DIETS FOR SPORTS PERFORMANCE: DID WE CALL THE 'NAIL IN THE COFFIN' TOO SOON?" SPORTS MED 45 SUPPL 1: S33-49.

51) MORRISON, P. F., ET AL. (2009). "THE INFLUENCE OF CONCURRENT ANTICONVULSANTS ON THE EFFICACY OF THE KETOGENIC DIET." EPILEPSIA 50(8): 1999-2001.

52) SMYL, C. (2016). "KETOGENIC DIET AND CANCER-A PERSPECTIVE." RECENT RESULTS CANCER RES 207: 233-240.

53) PAOLI, A. (2014). "KETOGENIC DIET FOR OBESITY: FRIEND OR FOE?" INT J ENVIRON RES PUBLIC HEALTH 11(2): 2092-2107.

54) PARTSALAKI, I., ET AL. (2012). "METABOLIC IMPACT OF A KETOGENIC DIET COMPARED TO A HYPOCALORIC DIET IN OBESE CHILDREN AND ADOLESCENTS." J PEDIATR ENDOCRINOL METAB 25(7-8): 697-704.

55) MAIORANA, A., ET AL. (2015). "KETOGENIC DIET IN A PATIENT WITH CONGENITAL HYPERINSULINISM: A NOVEL APPROACH TO PREVENT BRAIN DAMAGE." ORPHANET J RARE DIS 10: 120.

56) VEECH, R. L., ET AL. (2017). "KETONE BODIES MIMIC THE LIFE SPAN EXTENDING PROPERTIES OF CALORIC RESTRICTION." IUBMB LIFE 69(5): 305-314.

57) PAWLOSKY, R. J., ET AL. (2017). "EFFECTS OF A DIETARY KETONE ESTER ON HIPPOCAMPAL GLYCOLYTIC AND TRICARBOXYLIC ACID CYCLE INTERMEDIATES AND AMINO ACIDS IN A 3XTGAD MOUSE MODEL OF ALZHEIMER'S DISEASE." J NEUROCHEM 141(2): 195-207.

58) KEY, T. J., ET AL. (1998). "MORTALITY IN VEGETARIANS AND NON-VEGETARIANS: A COLLABORATIVE ANALYSIS OF 8300 DEATHS AMONG 76,000 MEN AND WOMEN IN FIVE PROSPECTIVE STUDIES." PUBLIC HEALTH NUTR 1(1): 33-41.

59) KEY, T. J., ET AL. (1999). "MORTALITY IN VEGETARIANS AND NONVEGETARIANS: DETAILED FINDINGS FROM A COLLABORATIVE ANALYSIS OF 5 PROSPECTIVE STUDIES." AM J CLIN NUTR 70(3 SUPPL): 516S-524S.

60) SINGH, S. P., ET AL. (2015). "RISK FACTORS ASSOCIATED WITH NON-ALCOHOLIC FATTY LIVER DISEASE IN INDIANS: A CASE-CONTROL STUDY." J CLIN EXP HEPATOL 5(4): 295-302.

61) MIHRSHAHI, S., ET AL. (2017). "VEGETARIAN DIET AND ALL-CAUSE MORTALITY: EVIDENCE FROM A LARGE POPULATION-BASED AUSTRALIAN COHORT - THE 45 AND UP STUDY." PREV MED 97: 1-7.

62) RAND, W. M., ET AL. (2003). "META-ANALYSIS OF NITROGEN BALANCE STUDIES FOR ESTIMATING PROTEIN REQUIREMENTS IN HEALTHY ADULTS." AM J CLIN NUTR 77(1): 109-127.

63) BLUM, M., ET AL. (1989). "PROTEIN INTAKE AND KIDNEY FUNCTION IN HUMANS: ITS EFFECT ON 'NORMAL AGING'." ARCH INTERN MED 149(1): 211-212.

64) WEIGLE, D. S., ET AL. (2005). "A HIGH-PROTEIN DIET INDUCES SUSTAINED REDUCTIONS IN APPETITE, AD LIBITUM CALORIC INTAKE, AND BODY WEIGHT DESPITE COMPENSATORY CHANGES IN DIURNAL PLASMA LEPTIN AND GHRELIN CONCENTRATIONS." AM J CLIN NUTR 82(1): 41-48.

65) INSTITUTE OF MEDICINE (E.-U.). (2005). DIETARY REFERENCE INTAKES FOR WATER, POTASSIUM, SODIUM, CHLORIDE, AND SULFATE. WASHINGTON, D.C: NATIONAL ACADEMIES PRESS: 456-459

66) SIMPSON, M. R. AND HOWARD, T. (2011). ACSM INFORMATION ON… SELECTING AND EFFECTIVELY USING HYDRATION FOR FITNESS.

67) LIEBER, C. S. (1997). "ETHANOL METABOLISM, CIRRHOSIS AND ALCOHOLISM." CLIN CHIM ACTA 257(1): 59-84.

68) LIEBER, C. S. (2000). "ALCOHOL: ITS METABOLISM AND INTERACTION WITH NUTRIENTS." ANNU REV NUTR 20: 395-430.

69) HILLER-STURMHOFEL, S. AND A. BARTKE (1998). "THE ENDOCRINE SYSTEM: AN OVERVIEW." ALCOHOL HEALTH RES WORLD 22(3): 153-164.

70) HATONEN, K. A., ET AL. (2012). "MODIFYING EFFECTS OF ALCOHOL ON THE POSTPRANDIAL GLUCOSE AND INSULIN RESPONSES IN HEALTHY SUBJECTS." AM J CLIN NUTR 96(1): 44-49.

71) Epstein, M. (1997). "Alcohol's impact on kidney function." Alcohol Health Res World 21(1): 84-92.

72) World, M. J., et al. (1985). "Alcoholic malnutrition and the small intestine." Alcohol Alcohol 20(2): 89-124.

73) Krasner, N., et al. (1976). "Alcohol and absorption from the small intestine. 1. Impairment of absorption from the small intestine in alcoholics." Gut 17(4): 245-248.

74) Chen, G., et al. (2012). "Autophagy is a protective response to ethanol neurotoxicity." Autophagy 8(11): 1577-1589.

75) Rubin, E., et al. (1976). "Prolonged ethanol consumption increases testosterone metabolism in the liver." Science 191(4227): 563-564.

76) Van Thiel, D. H., et al. (1975). "Alcohol-induced testicular atrophy. An experimental model for hypogonadism occurring in chronic alcoholic men." Gastroenterology 69(2): 326-332.

77) Mendelson, J. H., et al. (1988). "Acute alcohol effects on plasma estradiol levels in women." Psychopharmacology (Berl) 94(4): 464-467.

78) Coutelle, C., et al. (2004). "Risk factors in alcohol associated breast cancer: alcohol dehydrogenase polymorphism and estrogens." Int J Oncol 25(4): 1127-1132.

79) Lang, C. H., et al. (2003). "Alcohol impairs leucine-mediated phosphorylation of 4E-BP1, S6K1, eIF4G, and mTOR in skeletal muscle." Am J Physiol Endocrinol Metab 285(6): E1205-1215.

80) Di Minno, M. N., et al. (2011). "Alcohol dosing and the heart: updating clinical evidence." Semin Thromb Hemost 37(8): 875-884.

81) Queipo-Ortuno, M. I., et al. (2012). "Influence of red wine polyphenols and ethanol on the gut microbiota ecology and biochemical biomarkers." Am J Clin Nutr 95(6): 1323-1334.

82) Martin, B. C., et al. (1992). "Role of glucose and insulin resistance in development of type 2 diabetes mellitus: results of a 25-year follow-up study." Lancet 340(8825): 925-929.

83) Adimon, L., et al. (2012). "Atherosclerosis, platelets and thrombosis in acute ischaemic heart disease." Eur Heart J Acute Cardiovasc Care 1(1): 60-74.

84) Sacks, F. M., et al. (2014). "Effects of high vs low glycemic index of dietary carbohydrate on cardiovascular disease risk factors and insulin sensitivity: the OmniCarb randomized clinical trial." JAMA 312(23): 2531-2541.

85) Bray, G. A. (2008). "Fructose: should we worry?" Int J Obes (Lond) 32 Suppl 7: S127-131.

86) Melanson, K. J., et al. (2007). "Effects of high-fructose corn syrup and sucrose consumption on circulating glucose, insulin, leptin, and ghrelin and on appetite in normal-weight women." Nutrition 23(2): 103-112.

87) Stanhope, K. L. and P. J. Havel (2008). "Endocrine and metabolic effects of consuming beverages sweetened with fructose, glucose, sucrose, or high-fructose corn syrup." Am J Clin Nutr 88(6): 1733S-1737S.

88) DiNicolantonio, J. J. and A. Berger (2016). "Added sugars drive nutrient and energy deficit in obesity: a new paradigm." Open Heart 3(2): e000469.

89) BRAY, G. A., ET AL. (2004). "CONSUMPTION OF HIGH-FRUCTOSE CORN SYRUP IN BEVERAGES MAY PLAY A ROLE IN THE EPIDEMIC OF OBESITY." AM J CLIN NUTR 79(4): 537-543.

90) LALLES, J. P. (2016). "MICROBIOTA-HOST INTERPLAY AT THE GUT EPITHELIAL LEVEL, HEALTH AND NUTRITION." J ANIM SCI BIOTECHNOL 7: 66.

91) ROGERS, P. J. (2017). "FOOD AND DRUG ADDICTIONS: SIMILARITIES AND DIFFERENCES." PHARMACOL BIOCHEM BEHAV 153: 182-190.

92) AVENA, N. M., ET AL. (2008). "EVIDENCE FOR SUGAR ADDICTION: BEHAVIORAL AND NEUROCHEMICAL EFFECTS OF INTERMITTENT, EXCESSIVE SUGAR INTAKE." NEUROSCI BIOBEHAV REV 32(1): 20-39.

93) MERCER, M. E. AND M. D. HOLDER (1997). "FOOD CRAVINGS, ENDOGENOUS OPIOID PEPTIDES, AND FOOD INTAKE: A REVIEW." APPETITE 29(3): 325-352.

94) RATO, L., ET AL. (2013). "HIGH-ENERGY DIETS MAY INDUCE A PRE-DIABETIC STATE ALTERING TESTICULAR GLYCOLYTIC METABOLIC PROFILE AND MALE REPRODUCTIVE PARAMETERS." ANDROLOGY 1(3): 495-504.

95) VARZAKAS, T., ET AL. (2012). SWEETENERS: NUTRITIONAL ASPECTS, APPLICATIONS, AND PRODUCTION TECHNOLOGY, CRC PRESS. P.46-51.

96) BLAKE, J. S. (2016). NUTRITION & YOU, PEARSON. P.160-162.

97) CODE OF FEDERAL REGUALTIONS, TITLE 7, SUBTITILE B, CHAPTER I, SUBCHAPTER M, PART 205, SUBPART D, §205.301 PRODUCT COMPOSITION.

98) FOOD AND DRUG ADMINISTRATION (2013). A FOOD LABELING GUIDE: GUIDANCE FOR INDUSTRY. U.S. DEPARTMENT OF HEALTH AND HUMAN SERVICES. P. 87-90.

www.ingramcontent.com/pod-product-compliance
Lightning Source LLC
Chambersburg PA
CBHW020327290526
45785CB00007B/2950